YOGA FOR WOMEN OVER 40

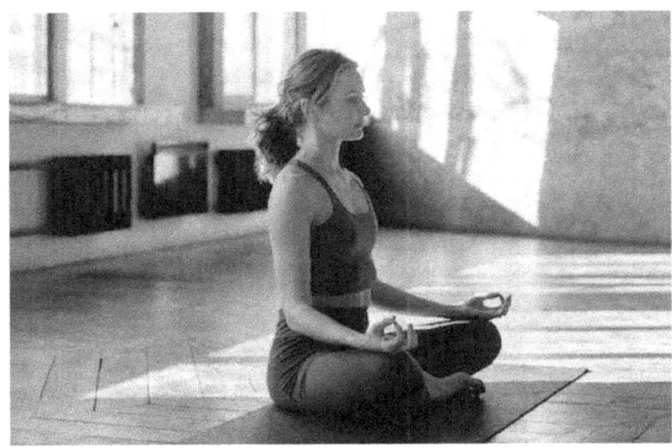

Dr. Kimberly Carlos

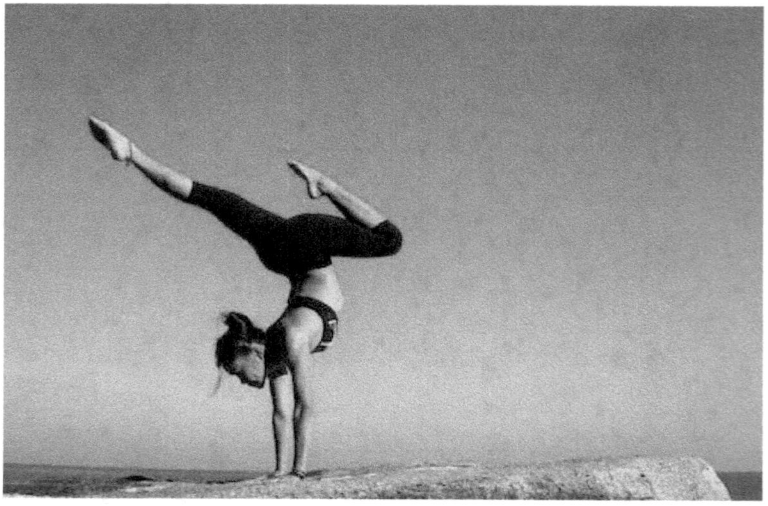

TABLE OF CONTENT

INTRODUCTION 7

CHAPTER ONE 11

How to Follow a Yoga for Women Over 40 Diet with Benefits 11

The Benefits of a Yoga Diet for Women Over 40 13

CHAPTER TWO 17

14 Day Yoga for Women Over 40 Diet Meal Plan........ 17

Day 1 17

Day 2 17

Day 3 18

Day 4 18

Day 5 19

Day 6 19

Day 7 20

Day 8 20

Day 9 21

Day 10 21

Day 11 22

Day 12 22

Day 13 23

Day 14 23

CHAPTER THREE 25

Yoga for Women Over 40 Exercises and How to Do Them
.... 25

1. Mountain Pose (Tadasana) 25

2. Downward-Facing Dog (Adho Mukha Svanasana).. 25

3. Warrior I (Virabhadrasana I) 25

4. Warrior II (Virabhadrasana II) 26

5. Warrior III (Virabhadrasana III) 26

6. Tree Pose (Vrksasana) 26

7. Bridge Pose (Setu Bandha Sarvangasana) 26

8. Cat-Cow Stretch (Marjaryasana/Bitilasana) 27

9. Child's Pose (Balasana) 27

10. Triangle Pose (Trikonasana) 27

11. Seated Forward Bend (Paschimottanasana) 27

12. Cobra Pose (Bhujangasana) 28

13. Sphinx Pose 28

14. Pigeon Pose (Eka Pada Rajakapotasana) 28

15. Extended Puppy Pose (Uttana Shishosana) 28

16. Extended Triangle Pose (Utthita Trikonasana) 29

17. Half Lord of the Fishes Pose (Ardha Matsyendrasana) 29

18. Legs-Up-the-Wall Pose (Viparita Karani) 29

19. Reclining Bound Angle Pose (Supta Baddha Konasana) 30

20. Happy Baby Pose (Ananda Balasana) 30

21. Supine Hand-to-Big-Toe Pose (Supta Padangusthasana) 30

22. Chair Pose (Utkatasana) 31

23. Plank Pose (Phalakasana) 31

24. Extended Hand-to-Big-Toe Pose (Utthita Hasta Padangusthasana) 31

25. Garland Pose (Malasana) 32

26. Camel Pose (Ustrasana) 32

27. Revolved Triangle Pose (Parivrtta Trikonasana) 32

28. Boat Pose (Navasana) 32

29. Sphinx Pose Variation 33

30. Legs-on-the-Chair Pose (Viparita Karani Variation) 33

31. Supported Bridge Pose 33

32. Dolphin Pose (Ardha Pincha Mayurasana) 33

33. Legs-Up-the-Wall Twist 34

34. Supported Shoulderstand (Salamba Sarvangasana Variation) 34

35. Sphinx Pose Variation 2 34

36. Supine Butterfly Pose (Supta Baddha Konasana Variation) 34

37. Happy Baby Twist 35

38. Supported Forward Fold 35

39. Lizard Pose (Utthan Pristhasana) 35

40. Restorative Savasana 35

CONCLUSION 37

INTRODUCTION

Once upon a time, in the quaint town of Serenity Springs, there lived a remarkable woman named Grace. Grace was a vibrant and spirited woman, full of life, but as she approached her 40s, she noticed her energy levels and flexibility weren't quite what they used to be.

Determined to reclaim her vitality, she decided to explore the world of yoga.

Grace had always been curious about yoga, but her busy life as a working mother had kept her from giving it a try. One day, while browsing the local community center's notice board, she noticed a flyer for a "Yoga for Women Over 40" class. It felt like fate, and she enrolled without hesitation.

The first day of class arrived, and Grace felt a mix of excitement and nervousness. She walked into the softly lit studio, where the soothing aroma of essential oils greeted her. The yoga instructor, Maya, welcomed her with a warm smile. Maya was a wise and experienced yogi, and she sensed Grace's apprehension.

With gentle encouragement, she assured Grace that this class was designed for women like her, embracing the wisdom and strength that comes with age.

As the weeks passed, Grace's passion for yoga blossomed. The carefully curated classes combined various yoga styles tailored to the needs of women over 40. Each session focused on building core strength, improving flexibility, and calming the mind.

Grace found that not only did her body grow stronger, but her mind also became clearer, more focused, and tranquil.

The other women in the class became her companions on this journey. They shared stories of triumphs and challenges, forming a supportive sisterhood that uplifted one another. Together, they learned to embrace their bodies with love and appreciation, understanding that age was a testament to their life experiences.

Beyond the physical benefits, yoga opened a new world for Grace. She began to explore mindfulness and meditation, which helped her find inner peace amidst life's chaos.

Her newfound serenity rippled into her daily life, improving her relationships with her family and friends.

One day, Grace noticed a poster for a regional yoga competition. At first, she dismissed the idea, thinking she wasn't skilled enough. But with Maya's encouragement and the unwavering support of her yoga sisters, Grace decided to participate.

The day of the competition arrived, and Grace took a deep breath as she stepped onto the stage. The audience watched in awe as she flowed through her poses with grace and confidence. Her performance was not about perfection; it was a testament to the journey she had undertaken – a celebration of embracing her true self.

As she finished her routine, the crowd erupted in applause. Grace felt a sense of accomplishment that went beyond any trophy or recognition. She had discovered her strength, not just in her body, but in her spirit.

Word of Grace's inspiring journey spread throughout Serenity Springs, and soon, more women over 40 flocked to Maya's yoga classes.

Grace's story became a beacon of hope and empowerment for all those who believed age was just a number.

And so, in this quaint town of Serenity Springs, the yoga studio became a hub of rejuvenation and self-discovery, all thanks to Grace's decision to embark on a transformative journey through yoga – a journey that proved age was not a barrier, but a stepping stone to a more fulfilled life.

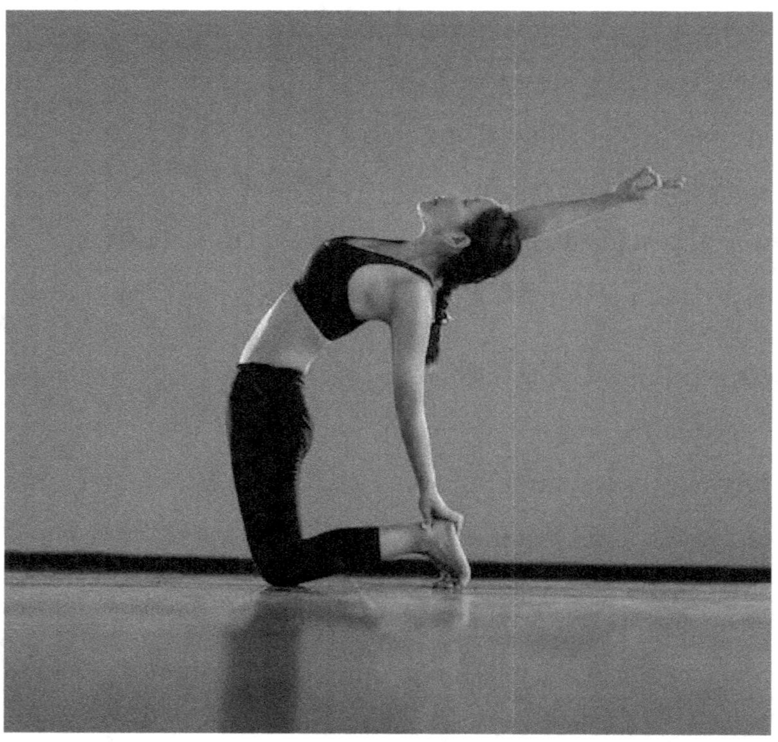

CHAPTER ONE

How to Follow a Yoga for Women Over 40 Diet with Benefits

As women reach their 40s and beyond, maintaining overall health and well-being becomes increasingly vital. In conjunction with regular yoga practice, adopting a suitable diet can help women over 40 feel energized, promote mental clarity, and support their bodies through the natural aging process. In this article, we will delve into the essential components of a Yoga diet for women over 40, its numerous health benefits, and practical tips to follow it effectively.

The Foundations of a Yoga Diet

1. Mindful Eating

Yoga promotes mindfulness, and the same approach should be applied to eating. Mindful eating involves savoring each bite, recognizing hunger and satiety cues, and being aware of the nutritional value of the food consumed. It also means cultivating a positive relationship with food and honoring the body's needs.

2. Emphasize Whole Foods

A Yoga diet centers around whole, unprocessed foods that are rich in nutrients. Opt for fresh fruits, vegetables, whole grains, nuts, seeds, lean proteins, and plant-based sources to fuel the body with essential vitamins, minerals, and antioxidants.

3. Hydration

Staying adequately hydrated is crucial for overall health and optimal yoga practice. Throughout the day, consume enough of water to promote digestion, increase energy, and preserve good skin.

4. Portion Control

As metabolism may slow down with age, it's essential to be mindful of portion sizes. Consuming balanced meals with appropriate portion control ensures a steady supply of energy without overloading the digestive system.

The Benefits of a Yoga Diet for Women Over 40

1. Increased Energy Levels

A nutrient-rich diet supports sustained energy levels throughout the day, enhancing one's ability to engage in daily activities, work, and yoga practice.

2. Enhanced Digestion

Whole foods are easier to digest and can help alleviate digestive issues commonly associated with aging, such as bloating and constipation.

3. Weight Management

Mindful eating and portion control can contribute to maintaining a healthy weight, reducing the risk of obesity-related health concerns.

4. Improved Mental Clarity

A well-balanced diet nourishes the brain and enhances cognitive function, promoting mental clarity, focus, and emotional balance.

5. Bone Health

For women over 40, bone health is of utmost importance. A diet rich in calcium and vitamin D, along with weight-bearing yoga postures, can support bone density and reduce the risk of osteoporosis.

6. Hormonal Balance

Certain whole foods, like flaxseeds and soy products, contain phytoestrogens that may help balance hormones during menopause.

7. Skin Radiance

The antioxidants present in fruits and vegetables help combat oxidative stress, promoting healthier, glowing skin.

Practical Tips for Following a Yoga Diet

1. Plan Balanced Meals

Prepare meals that are nutritionally diverse and well-balanced. Aim for a combination of complex carbohydrates, lean proteins, healthy fats, and ample fiber to support overall health.

2. Prioritize Breakfast

Start the day with a nourishing breakfast, which can stabilize blood sugar levels and provide sustained energy throughout the morning.

3. Snack Smartly

Choose nutrient-dense snacks like fresh fruits, nuts, or yogurt to curb hunger between meals.

4. Avoid Processed Foods

Minimize the consumption of processed and sugary foods as they offer little nutritional value and may lead to energy crashes.

5. Experiment with Plant-Based Meals

Explore vegetarian or vegan options for some of your meals, as plant-based diets have been associated with various health benefits.

6. Listen to Your Body

Pay attention to how certain foods make you feel. Every individual is unique, so adjust your diet based on how your body responds to different foods.

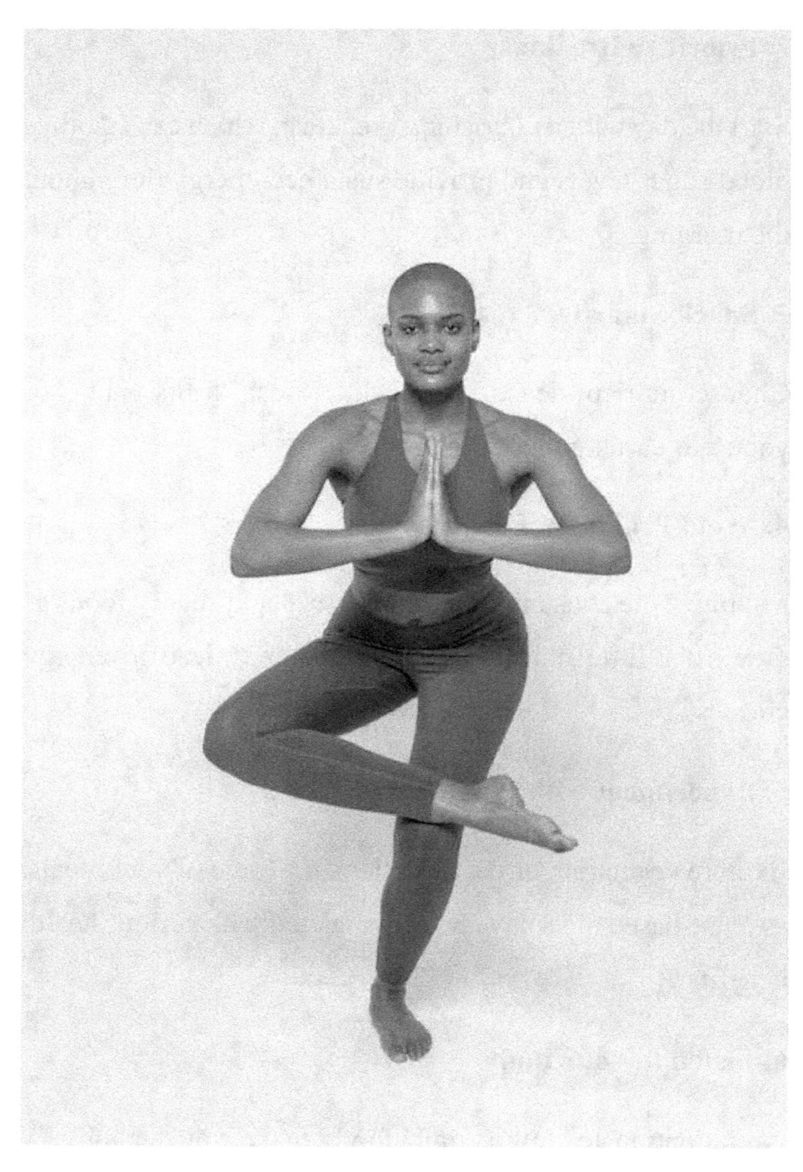

CHAPTER TWO

14 Day Yoga for Women Over 40 Diet Meal Plan

Day 1

- Breakfast: Greek yogurt topped with mixed berries, honey, and a sprinkle of chia seeds.
- Snack:Apple and a little handful of almonds.
- Lunch: Quinoa salad with roasted vegetables (bell peppers, zucchini, and cherry tomatoes) and a lemon-tahini dressing.
- Snack: Carrot sticks with hummus.
- Dinner: fish baked in the oven with quinoa and steam broccoli.

Day 2

- Breakfast: Smoothie made from almond milk, spinach, banana, and plant-based protein powder.
- Snack: Sliced cucumbers with a side of cottage cheese.
- Lunch: Lentil soup with a side of mixed greens and a lemon-olive oil dressing.
- Snack: Whole grain crackers with avocado slices.
- Dinner: Grilled chicken breast with asparagus and sweet potato.

Day 3

- Breakfast: Oatmeal topped with sliced peaches and a drizzle of maple syrup.
- Snack: Mixed nuts and a pear.
- Lunch: Brown rice stir-fry with tofu, broccoli, bell peppers, and a soy-ginger sauce.
- Snack: Sliced bell peppers with guacamole.
- Dinner: quinoa and baked cod with roasted Brussels sprouts.

Day 4

- Breakfast: Whole grain toast with avocado and poached eggs.
- Snack: Plain yogurt with a handful of mixed berries.
- Lunch: Chickpea salad with diced cucumbers, tomatoes, red onion, and a lemon-tahini dressing.
- Snack: Rice cakes with almond butter.
- Dinner: Grilled shrimp with a side of sautéed spinach and brown rice.

Day 5

- Breakfast: Chia seed pudding with coconut milk and sliced kiwi.
- Snack: Celery sticks with peanut butter.
- Lunch: Spinach and feta stuffed bell peppers with a side of quinoa.
- Snack: Orange slices and a handful of walnuts.
- Dinner: roasted sweet potato, roasted green beans, and baked chicken.

Day 6

- Breakfast: Smoothie with kale, pineapple, banana, and coconut water.
- Snack: Cottage cheese with pineapple chunks.
- Lunch: Mixed bean salad with tomatoes, corn, and cilantro-lime dressing.
- Snack: Rice cakes with sliced avocado.
- Dinner: Grilled steak with a side of asparagus and mashed cauliflower.

Day 7

- Breakfast: Overnight oats with almond milk, sliced strawberries, and a drizzle of honey.
- Snack: Sliced mango and a handful of cashews.
- Lunch: Black bean and quinoa-stuffed bell peppers.
- Snack: Sliced cucumbers with tzatziki sauce.
- Dinner: quinoa and baked tilapia with broccoli.

Day 8

- Breakfast: Greek yogurt topped with mixed berries, honey, and a sprinkle of chia seeds.
- Snack: Apple and a little handful of almonds.
- Lunch: Quinoa salad with roasted vegetables (bell peppers, zucchini, and cherry tomatoes) and a lemon-tahini dressing.
- Snack: Carrot sticks with hummus.
- Dinner: fish baked in the oven with quinoa and steam broccoli.

Day 9

- Breakfast: Smoothie made from almond milk, spinach, banana, and plant-based protein powder.
- Snack: Sliced cucumbers with a side of cottage cheese.
- Lunch: Lentil soup with a side of mixed greens and a lemon-olive oil dressing.
- Snack: Whole grain crackers with avocado slices.
- Dinner: Grilled chicken breast with asparagus and sweet potato.

Day 10

- Breakfast: Oatmeal topped with sliced peaches and a drizzle of maple syrup.
- Snack: Mixed nuts and a pear.
- Lunch: Brown rice stir-fry with tofu, broccoli, bell peppers, and a soy-ginger sauce.
- Snack: Sliced bell peppers with guacamole.
- Dinner: quinoa and baked cod with roasted Brussels sprouts.

Day 11

- Breakfast: Whole grain toast with avocado and poached eggs.
- Snack: Plain yogurt with a handful of mixed berries.
- Lunch: Chickpea salad with diced cucumbers, tomatoes, red onion, and a lemon-tahini dressing.
- Snack: Rice cakes with almond butter.
- Dinner: Grilled shrimp with a side of sautéed spinach and brown rice.

Day 12

- Breakfast: Chia seed pudding with coconut milk and sliced kiwi.
- Snack: Celery sticks with peanut butter.
- Lunch: Spinach and feta stuffed bell peppers with a side of quinoa.
- Snack: Orange slices and a handful of walnuts.
- Dinner: roasted sweet potato, roasted green beans, and baked chicken.

Day 13

- Breakfast: Smoothie with kale, pineapple, banana, and coconut water.
- Snack: Cottage cheese with pineapple chunks.
- Lunch: Mixed bean salad with tomatoes, corn, and cilantro-lime dressing.
- Snack: Rice cakes with sliced avocado.
- Dinner: Grilled steak with a side of asparagus and mashed cauliflower.

Day 14

- Breakfast: Overnight oats with almond milk, sliced strawberries, and a drizzle of honey.
- Snack: Sliced mango and a handful of cashews.
- Lunch: Black bean and quinoa-stuffed bell peppers.
- Snack: Sliced cucumbers with tzatziki sauce.
- Dinner: quinoa and baked tilapia with broccoli.

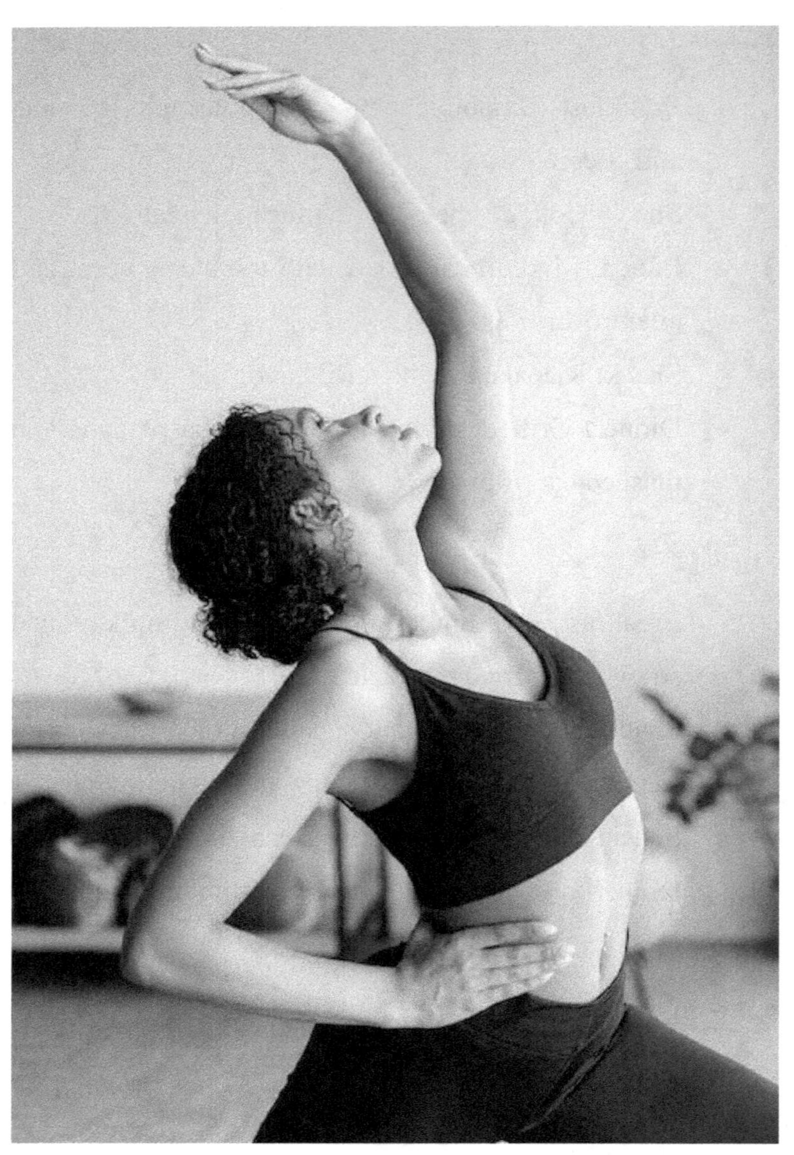

CHAPTER THREE

Yoga for Women Over 40 Exercises and How to Do Them

1. Mountain Pose (Tadasana)

- Stand tall with feet hip-width apart, arms at your sides, palms facing forward.
- Squeeze your abs and relax your shoulders. Lengthen your spine.

2. Downward-Facing Dog (Adho Mukha Svanasana)

- Start on hands and knees, lift hips to form an inverted V.
- Press hands and heels down, relax your head between your arms.

3. Warrior I (Virabhadrasana I)

Step one foot forward, bend front knee, back foot turned slightly out.

Raise arms overhead, gaze forward, and sink into your hips.

4. Warrior II (Virabhadrasana II)

- Extend arms parallel to the floor, front knee bent, back leg straight.
- Gaze over the front hand, aligning it with the bent knee.

5. Warrior III (Virabhadrasana III)

- Balance on one leg, extend opposite leg back, parallel to the ground.
- Reach arms forward, engage your core for balance.

6. Tree Pose (Vrksasana)

- Put your weight on one leg and rest the sole of your other foot on your inner thigh or calf.
- Hands can be at your heart center or raised overhead.

7. Bridge Pose (Setu Bandha Sarvangasana)

- Lie on your back, bend knees, place feet hip-width apart.
- Press into feet, lift hips, and interlace fingers beneath your back.

8. Cat-Cow Stretch (Marjaryasana/Bitilasana)

- Start on hands and knees, arch your back on the inhale, round it on the exhale.
- Move in sync with your breath, gently massaging the spine.

9. Child's Pose (Balasana)

- Kneel, sit back on heels, extend arms forward.
- Rest forehead on the ground, relax into the stretch.

10. Triangle Pose (Trikonasana)

- Stand with legs wide apart, reach one arm down and opposite arm up.
- Extend from the hips, hinge at the side waist, and look up at the raised hand.

11. Seated Forward Bend (Paschimottanasana)

- Sit upright and flex your feet.
- Hinge at hips, reach for your feet or shins, lengthening your spine.

12. Cobra Pose (Bhujangasana)

- Lie on your belly, place palms under shoulders.
- Inhale, press into hands, lift your chest, and arch your back.

13. Sphinx Pose

- Lie on your belly, prop up on your forearms, keeping elbows under shoulders.
- Press forearms down, lift chest, and lengthen your spine.

14. Pigeon Pose (Eka Pada Rajakapotasana)

- Start in a plank, bring one knee towards your hands, lower hips and extend back leg.
- Square hips and fold over the front leg, allowing a gentle hip stretch.

15. Extended Puppy Pose (Uttana Shishosana)

- Start on hands and knees, walk hands forward while keeping hips above knees.
- Lower your chest towards the ground, relaxing into a gentle stretch.

16. Extended Triangle Pose (Utthita Trikonasana)

- From Warrior II, straighten front leg and reach forward with one arm.
- Hinge at the hips, keeping legs straight, and other arm reaching up.

17. Half Lord of the Fishes Pose (Ardha Matsyendrasana)

- Sit with legs extended, bend one knee and place foot outside the opposite thigh.
- Twist towards the bent knee, placing opposite elbow outside the knee.

18. Legs-Up-the-Wall Pose (Viparita Karani)

- Lie on your back near a wall, extend legs up the wall.
- Relax arms at your sides, stay for a calming inversion.

19. Reclining Bound Angle Pose (Supta Baddha Konasana)

- Lie on your back, bring soles of feet together, let knees drop to the sides.
- Relax arms on the ground, allowing hips to gently open.

20. Happy Baby Pose (Ananda Balasana)

- Lie on your back, grab the outer edges of your feet, and bend knees towards your armpits.
- Gently rock side to side, feeling a hip and groin stretch.

21. Supine Hand-to-Big-Toe Pose (Supta Padangusthasana)

- Lie on your back, extend one leg up towards the ceiling, holding the big toe.
- Keep the other leg extended on the ground, gently pulling the raised leg closer.

22. Chair Pose (Utkatasana)

- Stand with feet together, bend knees as if sitting in an imaginary chair.
- Raise arms overhead or keep them at heart center, engaging your core.

23. Plank Pose (Phalakasana)

- Start in a push-up position, align wrists under shoulders.
- Maintain a straight line from head to heels while engaging your core.

24. Extended Hand-to-Big-Toe Pose (Utthita Hasta Padangusthasana)

- Stand, lift one leg forward, hold the big toe with the same-side hand.
- Straighten the leg out in front, engaging your core for balance.

25. Garland Pose (Malasana)

-   Squat down with feet slightly wider than hip-width, toes pointing outward.
-   Bring palms together at your heart center, using elbows to gently push knees apart.

26. Camel Pose (Ustrasana)

-   Kneel, tuck toes under, reach back to hold heels.
-   Lift chest, arch back, and gently drop your head behind.

27. Revolved Triangle Pose (Parivrtta Trikonasana)

-   From Extended Triangle Pose, twist your torso to one side.
-   Place the hand on the ground or a block, extend the opposite arm up.

28. Boat Pose (Navasana)

-   Sit on the ground, lift legs off the ground to form a V-shape.
-   Keep your back straight, balancing on your sitting bones, engage your core.

29. Sphinx Pose Variation

- Lie on your belly, prop up on your forearms, elbows under shoulders.
- Slide one arm forward, allowing a gentle twist and stretch through the spine.

30. Legs-on-the-Chair Pose (Viparita Karani Variation)

- Sit on the ground with legs extended, place feet on a chair seat.
- Rest your upper body on the ground, allowing for a gentle inversion.

31. Supported Bridge Pose

- Lie on your back, place a block or cushion under your sacrum.
- Relax hips on the support, allowing a gentle chest opening.

32. Dolphin Pose (Ardha Pincha Mayurasana)

- Start on forearms and knees, lift hips towards the ceiling.
- Keep your head off the ground, forming an inverted V shape.

33. Legs-Up-the-Wall Twist

- Lie on your back near a wall, extend legs up the wall.

- Gently drop legs to one side, twist your upper body in the opposite direction.

34. Supported Shoulderstand (Salamba Sarvangasana Variation)

- Lie on your back, lift legs up towards the ceiling.

- Place your hands on your lower back for support, forming a straight line from head to feet.

35. Sphinx Pose Variation 2

- Lie on your belly, prop up on your forearms, elbows under shoulders.

- Lift your upper body, bringing your chest off the ground, creating a deeper backbend.

36. Supine Butterfly Pose (Supta Baddha Konasana Variation)

- Lie on your back, bring the soles of your feet together.

- Allow your knees to gently drop to the sides, feeling a hip and groin stretch.

37. Happy Baby Twist

- Lie on your back, bend knees towards armpits, hold the outer edges of your feet.
- Gently drop your knees to one side, creating a twist while feeling a hip stretch.

38. Supported Forward Fold

- Sit with legs extended, place a cushion or bolster on your legs.
- Fold forward, allowing your upper body to rest on the support.

39. Lizard Pose (Utthan Pristhasana)

- From a lunge position, lower one forearm to the ground inside your front foot.
- Keep the back leg extended, gently sinking into the hips for a hip flexor stretch.

40. Restorative Savasana

- Lie on your back, arrange props like cushions or blankets for support.
- Relax your entire body, allowing yourself to fully surrender and rejuvenate.

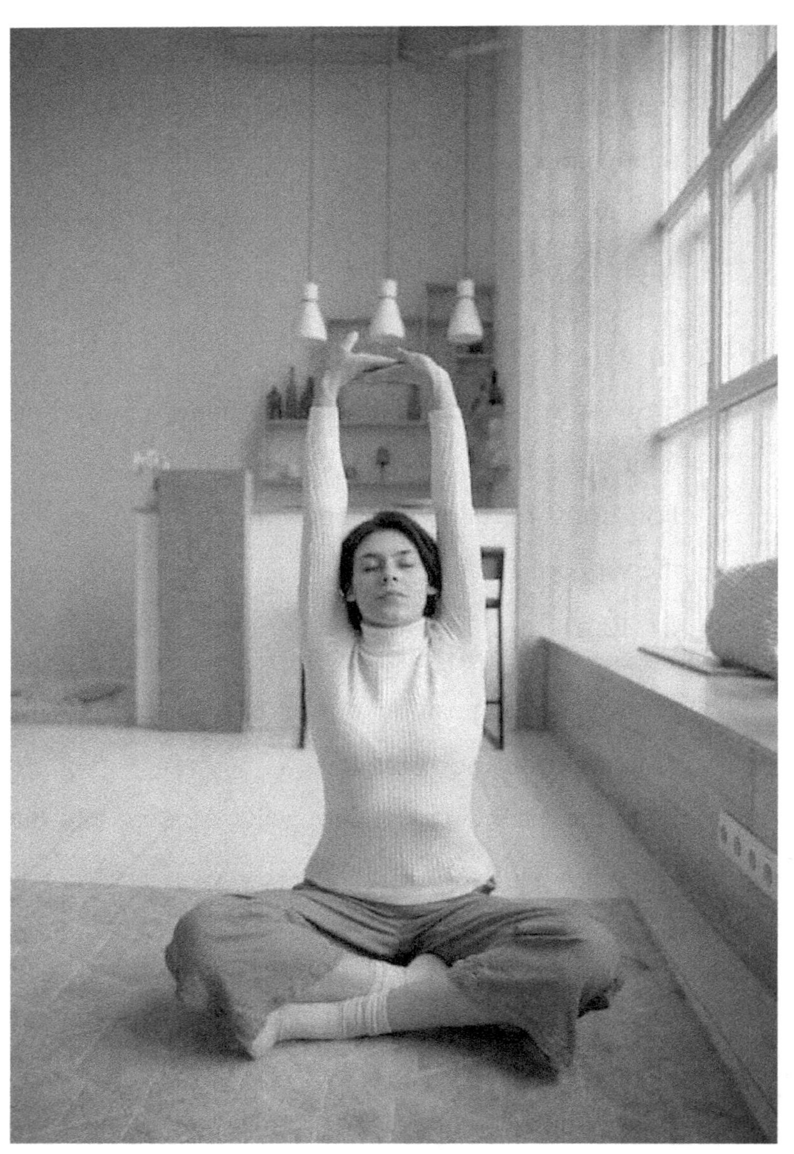

CONCLUSION

In conclusion, yoga is an invaluable practice for women over 40, offering a multitude of physical, mental, and emotional benefits. As women enter this stage of life, they may face unique challenges related to hormonal changes, decreased bone density, stress, and overall well-being.

Fortunately, yoga serves as a holistic and accessible solution to address these concerns and enhance their quality of life.

Physically, yoga provides a gentle yet effective way to maintain and improve flexibility, strength, and balance. With age, muscles and joints may become stiffer, leading to discomfort and limited mobility.

Through regular yoga practice, women can counteract these effects by stretching and strengthening their muscles, enhancing joint mobility, and promoting better posture.

Moreover, weight-bearing yoga postures contribute to maintaining bone density and reducing the risk of osteoporosis, a crucial consideration for women in this age group.

Mentally and emotionally, yoga offers a sanctuary for self-reflection, relaxation, and stress reduction. The meditative aspects of yoga allow women over 40 to find inner peace, reduce anxiety, and cultivate a positive outlook on life.

Mindfulness practices in yoga encourage women to stay present in the moment, fostering a deeper connection with their bodies and emotions. As they navigate life's changes, yoga equips them with tools to cope with stress, boost their mental clarity, and enhance overall emotional well-being.

Beyond the physical and mental benefits, yoga for women over 40 fosters a sense of community and empowerment. Attending yoga classes provides an opportunity for social engagement, connecting women with others who share similar experiences and goals.

The support and camaraderie found in yoga studios create a nurturing environment, where women can feel inspired and encouraged in their journey towards better health and self-discovery.

The adaptability of yoga makes it a truly inclusive practice for women of all ages, shapes, and fitness levels.

Whether a woman is new to yoga or a seasoned practitioner, there are modifications and variations that suit individual needs. This inclusivity allows women over 40 to tailor their yoga practice to suit their bodies and goals, ensuring a safe and effective experience.

Furthermore, yoga for women over 40 is not just a fitness regimen; it is a holistic approach to overall well-being. The combination of physical movement, breathwork, and mindfulness fosters harmony between the body, mind, and spirit.

As women embrace this holistic approach, they find themselves better equipped to navigate the challenges and changes that come with aging gracefully.

As with any fitness or wellness practice, it is essential for women over 40 to approach yoga with self-compassion and patience. Results may not be immediate, but with consistent practice, they will experience the transformative effects of yoga over time. Seeking guidance from experienced yoga instructors and healthcare professionals can help women tailor their practice to suit their unique needs and address any specific health concerns.

In conclusion, yoga serves as a powerful and accessible tool for women over 40 to maintain physical health, find mental clarity, and cultivate emotional well-being. Its gentle yet profound impact extends far beyond the mat, enriching every aspect of a woman's life.

Embracing yoga as a lifestyle offers a path towards self-discovery, empowerment, and a renewed sense of vitality, making the journey through life's later stages a fulfilling and transformative experience. Through yoga, women over 40 can embark on a lifelong journey of self-care, self-awareness, and inner growth, embracing each moment with grace and gratitude.

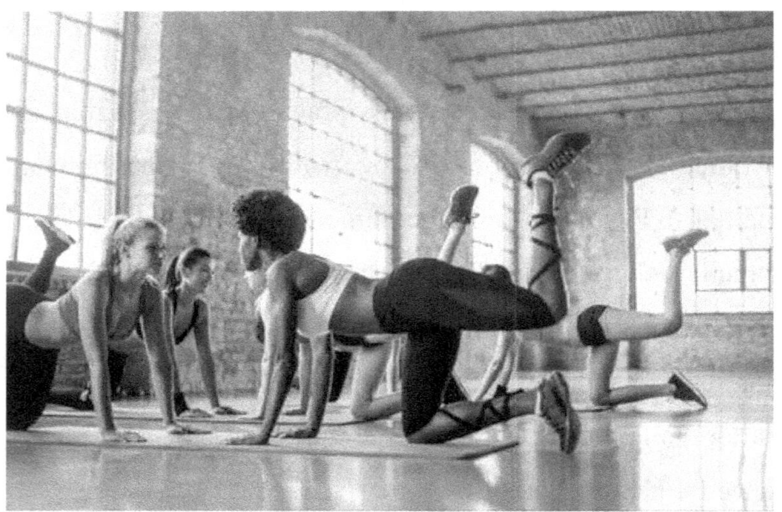

www.ingramcontent.com/pod-product-compliance
Lightning Source LLC
Chambersburg PA
CBHW071002250726
48663CB00002B/350

SUMÁRIO

APRESENTAÇÃO

CAPÍTULO I - INTRODUÇÃO À IMUNIDADE TRIBUTÁRIA
- O que é imunidade tributária?
- Diferença entre imunidade e isenção.
- Importância da imunidade tributária para os cidadãos.

CAPÍTULO II - PRINCÍPIOS CONSTITUCIONAIS
- Princípio da legalidade.
- Princípio da isonomia.
- Outros princípios relacionados à imunidade.

CAPÍTULO III - IMUNIDADE TRIBUTÁRIA RELIGIOSA
- Imunidade tributária para templos religiosos.
- Requisitos e limitações para usufruir da imunidade religiosa.
- Possíveis questionamentos e casos polêmicos.

CAPÍTULO VI - IMUNIDADE TRIBUTÁRIA CULTURAL
- Imunidade tributária para instituições culturais.
- Benefícios da imunidade para o desenvolvimento cultural do país.
- Como comprovar a finalidade cultural e garantir a imunidade.

CAPÍTULO V - IMUNIDADE TRIBUTÁRIA EDUCACIONAL
- Imunidade tributária para instituições de ensino.
- Abordagem das imunidades para diferentes níveis de ensino.
- Documentação e exigências para usufruir da imunidade educacional.

CAPÍTULO VI - IMUNIDADE TRIBUTÁRIA DE ENTIDADES FILANTRÓPICAS
- Imunidade tributária para entidades sem fins lucrativos.
- Critérios e requisitos para obter a imunidade filantrópica.
- Benefícios e obrigações das instituições filantrópicas.

CAPÍTULO VII – IMUNIDADE TRIBUTÁRIA DE EXPORTAÇÕES
- Imunidade tributária para produtos destinados à exportação.
- Como as empresas podem se beneficiar dessa imunidade.
- Limitações e exceções relacionadas à imunidade de exportações.

CAPÍTULO VIII – IMUNIDADE TRIBUTÁRIA AMBIENTAL
- Imunidade tributária para atividades relacionadas ao meio ambiente.
- Exemplos de setores e práticas que podem usufruir da imunidade ambiental.
- Compromissos e responsabilidades das empresas beneficiadas.

CAPÍTULO XI – LIMITAÇÕES E RESTRIÇÕES DA IMUNIDADE TRIBUTÁRIA
- Situações em que a imunidade tributária pode ser questionada.
- Exceções e limitações impostas pela legislação.
- Jurisprudências relevantes sobre limitações da imunidade.

CAPÍTULO X – ORIENTAÇÕES PRÁTICAS PARA GARANTIR SEUS DIREITOS
- Documentação necessária para comprovar a imunidade tributária.
- Procedimentos para obter o reconhecimento da imunidade.
- Recursos e medidas em caso de questionamentos ou negativas.

CONCLUSÃO: PROTEGENDO SEUS DIREITOS E CONTRIBUINDO PARA UMA SOCIEDADE JUSTA
- A importância da conscientização sobre os direitos de imunidade tributária.
- Como garantir o cumprimento dos seus direitos e colaborar para uma sociedade mais justa.

BIBLIOGRAFIA

APRESENTAÇÃO

VOCÊ JÁ OUVIU FALAR EM IMUNIDADE TRIBUTÁRIA? SABE QUAIS SÃO OS DIREITOS, GARANTIAS E OBRIGAÇÕES E COMO GARANTIR QUE SEJAM RESPEITADOS?

Se essas questões despertam o seu interesse e você deseja compreender melhor esse tema complexo, temos o prazer de apresentar o ebook "Imunidade Tributária Descomplicada: Guia Prático para Entender seus Direitos".

Neste guia abrangente e acessível, mergulharemos no mundo da imunidade tributária e exploraremos os diversos aspectos que envolvem esse assunto tão relevante para a sociedade. Ao longo de seus 10 capítulos, vamos desvendar os princípios, requisitos, limitações e benefícios relacionados às imunidades tributárias em diferentes áreas.

Este ebook foi cuidadosamente elaborado para trazer clareza e orientação sobre a imunidade tributária, de forma acessível e descomplicada. Nossa intenção é fornecer a você, leitor, as ferramentas necessárias para compreender seus direitos, proteger-se e contribuir para uma sociedade mais justa.

A imunidade tributária é um tema de relevância inegável, e seu entendimento é fundamental para o exercício pleno dos nossos direitos e para a promoção de um ambiente socioeconômico equitativo. Convidamos você a embarcar nessa jornada de conhecimento e descoberta, desvendando os segredos da imunidade tributária e fortalecendo sua posição na busca pela justiça fiscal.

Estamos aqui para auxiliá-lo nessa jornada e capacitá-lo a proteger seus direitos e contribuir para uma sociedade mais justa e igualitária.

Desejamos uma excelente e prazerosa leitura!!

CAPÍTULO I

INTRODUÇÃO À IMUNIDADE TRIBUTÁRIA

No primeiro capítulo deste ebook, vamos apresentar o instituto da imunidade tributária. Você provavelmente já ouviu falar sobre esse termo, mas pode não estar totalmente familiarizado com seu significado e importância.

O que é imunidade tributária?
Em termos simples, é um direito garantido pela Constituição que isenta determinadas pessoas, entidades ou atividades do pagamento de impostos. Isso significa que existem certas situações em que o Estado não pode cobrar tributos, mesmo que estejam previstos na legislação.

Diferença entre imunidade e isenção.
É fundamental compreender a diferença entre imunidade e isenção tributária. Enquanto a imunidade é uma garantia constitucional que não pode ser revogada pelo poder legislativo, a isenção é uma concessão legal que pode ser alterada ou revogada a qualquer momento.

Importância da imunidade tributária para os cidadãos.
A imunidade tributária desempenha um papel crucial na proteção dos direitos e garantias individuais. Ela está ancorada em princípios constitucionais, como o da legalidade, que estabelece que nenhum tributo pode ser cobrado sem previsão em lei. Além disso, a imunidade também está relacionada ao princípio da isonomia, que busca tratar igualmente aqueles que se encontram em situações semelhantes.

Ao compreendermos a imunidade tributária, percebemos sua importância para os cidadãos. Ela promove a liberdade de culto, garantindo que as instituições religiosas não sejam sobrecarregadas com impostos, e incentiva o desenvolvimento cultural e educacional, protegendo as entidades que se dedicam a essas áreas.